The Midwife in Me

Jane Blyth

This book is dedicated to my amazing family, the colleagues I have worked with and of course, the women and families whose experiences in childbirth, brought out "The Midwife in Me".

CONTENTS

INTRODUCTION

I have written this book about my journey to become a midwife and to share some of the many memories of my career, with my family and friends who have been with me along the way and to you the reader, an insight into the wonder of childbirth and the role of a Midwife.

I hope my book will inspire anyone considering joining the midwifery profession, to explore the opportunities and start their own journey. I wish them the fulfilment I found from this most rewarding role.

I have had some amazing experiences throughout my twenty-three years in midwifery. I cannot mention them all, but every birth played an important part in making me the midwife I became and contributed towards the satisfaction I have found from a career which has resulted in me feeling eternally blessed.

A midwife's role is to care for the mother, the unborn child and all those associated with them. The experience of being with women and their families, during their most vulnerable and life changing experience, of bringing new life into the world is such a privilege.

My aim was always to ensure I had provided the best care to my women, enabling a woman and her family to feel informed, supported and have the most positive experience possible.

At the end of the day, babies will be born anywhere regardless of the situation the mother finds herself in.

Over the years, as with many things there have been changes in Midwifery practice. I have seen a lot in my career and although the aim of progress and change is to optimise the overall outcome, sometimes we discover that some of the original ways were better for the mother and baby, and these can now be considered in best practice.

WHY MIDWIFERY?

I was the second child and although I was very excited about having a baby sister who was born when I was eight, I was not able to be involved much with her. She had rhesus incompatibility and was very ill at birth requiring a blood exchange transfusion. Not only did this make everyone very nervous about caring for her but I was regarded as a tomboy who couldn't be trusted with a baby. My clearest memory of the day she was born was that my sister and I were given a glass of Tizer, (a fizzy drink), and a bag of crisps to celebrate her arrival.

From a young age I had a love of babies and could not resist the opportunity to look after a baby. As I got older, I was entrusted with other people's babies, whether it was staying with a cousin helping her when she had her first baby or caring for a neighbour's baby, taking her out for walks in her super shiny bassinette pram.

What influenced my decision to become a nurse?

Was it my mother coming home after a night shift, as an auxiliary nurse (now known as a maternity assistant)? She worked in a maternity unit and often shared her experiences with me over breakfast.

I remember her telling me about caesarean sections. In those days, the blood-soaked swabs were thrown on the floor and her role involved picking them up and hang them on a counting rail. If she wasn't quick enough, she would be hit by the next one.

Was it working as a teenager, in the same maternity unit as my mother serving the teas at weekends? In those days each woman had her own tray, teapot, milk jug, sugar bowl and cup and saucer. After serving the teas my job included washing these up by hand as there was no dishwasher then.

Was it working on the neonatal unit as a general cleaner? A temporary job after leaving school before commencing my nurse training. Although I had nothing to do with the babies, I still had to wear a gown over my cleaner's uniform as the unit had to be kept infection free. Only the nurses could clean any equipment used by or for the babies. My time there gave me valuable insight, into the amazing work of caring for new life. I remember the patience of one doctor, spending two hours putting in an intravenous line (a means of gaining direct access to the baby's circulation for giving medication) into a very sick baby's arm.

This was where I started learning the importance of hygiene measures in the prevention of cross infection.

I also observed the ups and downs of caring for sick babies and learned more about the sensitivity required to care for their families during both the good and difficult times. Most importantly, I grew up quickly.

I was fortunate to know what I wanted to do when I left school, which was to become a nurse. I was impatient and did not want to wait until I was eighteen, the usual age to start nursing training. This led me to apply to the Royal National Orthopaedic Hospital (RNOH) to be an Orthopaedic Nursing student, which in 1968, you could start at seventeen.

Once accepted and without a second thought, I moved away from my home in Sussex and headed to the hustle and bustle of London to commence my career in nursing. The Royal National Orthopaedic Hospital is in Stanmore, North London, but still a far cry from my home and the place I had known since the age of six.

THE HAND OF FATE

It was at this point that my life almost took another path. One which could have been so different to the one I am sharing with you now.

I had moved into the nursing home, collected my uniforms and was in the first week of my initial study block. I was intently listening to a lecture on bandaging, when I became aware of a disturbance in the doorway and a senior tutor came in clutching a piece of paper.

It became obvious that she needed to interrupt the lecture and seized her opportunity when we reached a break in the session. I must admit to feeling distracted, wondering what her message was to be.

Little did I know that it was to be directed at me. Clearing her throat, she looked around the classroom, scanning for my presence before calling out, "Jane Wilson. Would you please follow me to reception?" I had been called from the lecture to be told that there had been an error in the acceptance of my qualifications to train at the RNOH.

The requirement was five 'O' levels or the entrance exam. The RNOH were only offering places to those with a minimum of five 'O' levels, and I only had two! They were most apologetic and offered me the opportunity to sit the entrance exam as the error had occurred within their administration department. With no time to prepare and still reeling from the devastating news that I may have to cease training, I was informed that I would need to sit the entrance exam immediately and if I was not successful, I would have to leave.

I did not have a choice. I was led to a room where I nervously sat the exam and prayed that I would be successful and pass. Thankfully I did and was allowed to continue my training, which after two years I duly qualified and gained my State Orthopaedic Nursing Certificate.

Occasionally, I wonder what might have become of me if I had not passed the entrance exam that day.

Would I have, persevered, taken evening classes, or waited until I was eighteen to fulfil my destiny?

Would I have met my husband and be where I am today?

MY DREAMS

Along with wanting to become a nurse, I hoped one day to fall in love, get married and have a family of my own.

It was towards the end of my orthopaedic training at the RNOH that I met my future husband. Graham was a member of the rugby club situated next to the hospital and unsurprisingly this was where the nurses could be found socialising most weekends.

One night in January, he walked me home for the first time and on the steps of the nursing home he went to kiss me goodnight. I was horrified and stopped him, telling him that his face was too rough and unshaven. Apparently, this was a prerequisite for a front row rugby prop, to be as unpleasant as possible when scrumming down with the opposition. He went home, shaved, and returned for that first kiss which I accepted gracefully. I then said "goodnight" and sent him home, hoping he would contact me again!

Life in those days was very different from today, men were not allowed in the Nurse's Home and the doors were locked at 10pm.

On reflection, our relationship could have ended there but luckily it progressed and looking back, that was a special moment in our future together. Our relationship grew and we went on to make plans to marry the following year.

It might sound old fashioned to the generation of today, but marriage was a role I took very seriously, and I wanted to be a good wife.

At this point and to have time to plan my wedding and future with Graham, I did not continue with my general training. I decided to move back to my family home in Sussex until the wedding, leaving Graham behind. I became a Ground Hostess for Caledonian Airways at Gatwick Airport, commuting to see him every week.

Luckily, I had to have my tonsils out during that time and being back in a hospital made me realise I really wanted to continue and become a nurse.

I quickly applied for Enrolled Nurse training at Crawley Hospital, I was accepted, and started training.

I opted to undertake the shortened course of general training, to become a State Enrolled Nurse (SEN), to ensure I could finish the training and manage my career along with the role of being a wife and building a home with my husband.

I missed Graham while living at home, so transferred back to the newly opened Northwick Park Hospital (NPH), in Harrow, to be closer to him and continue my training. My cohort were the first pupil nurses to train there. Rules were much more relaxed and to my surprise he was allowed into my room, although not allowed to stay overnight.

Graham and I were married in 1971, just after I qualified and we set up home in Wembley.

Throughout my training as a nurse, I always gravitated to the children's wards, spending time with the babies and toddlers whose parents, lived a long way away and were unable to visit regularly. In my off-duty time I would often babysit locally as like many of the other nurses, we all needed a little extra to top up our wages.

I looked to continue my nursing career by fulfilling my early dreams of working with new life and becoming a midwife. I transferred to the maternity unit at Northwick Park Hospital, as a State Enrolled Nurse to find out if this was the right path for me.

It was not long before I found myself pregnant and commenced my most fulfilling role ever, becoming a mother.

BECOMING A MOTHER

Although not a planned pregnancy, I was so excited to have this new life growing inside me. Being pregnant and giving birth three times were my most amazing experiences in life and my best achievements by far.

I remained at home for several years when I very much enjoyed being with my children. My second daughter had several health issues and needed to be hospitalised on numerous occasions. I was in a fortunate position to be able to be with her all that time. I only went back to work two evenings a week initially, when my last daughter was eighteen months old.

I was booked to have my first baby in Northwick Park Hospital. I had spent some time on the delivery suite in my general training and having worked in the maternity unit until leaving to have my baby, I had met most of the staff. All the midwives were lovely and there was only one I was a little unsure of, so when wondering who might attend my delivery, there was only one midwife I hoped I would not get in labour.

You can imagine my anxiety when I was greeted by you guessed it, the very same midwife. How wrong my impression of her had been, she was so caring and made me feel safe.

This turned out to be a valuable learning experience I would carry with me in my future practice, not to pre-judge anyone.

My first birth was induced due to post maturity, that is not reference to my age but the fact that I was two weeks overdue. I arrived on the delivery suite, looking good, I thought, I had even curled my hair! I might not have bothered if I had known what was to come.

I was shaved and given an enema to empty my bowels as was the protocol for birthing preparation then. After a short while I started to feel some very uncomfortable sensations and was surprised that things were happening so quickly. I remember thinking, this is it, I'm about to give birth. You can imagine my disappointment when the midwife informed me it was just the enema working!

Next, I was taken to a large theatre like room and told to lie on the bed and my legs were put up and supported in stirrups. The consultant obstetrician came into the room and proceeded to break my waters with an instrument that looked like something my Granny used to crochet with. The implement felt it was about to emerge through my throat, which obviously it was not. I then felt a warmness draining from me, I was given a pad between my legs and advised to walk around along with a drip stand on wheels. I felt then that all my dignity was gone. The drip contained a drug to start my contractions.

I did not need to be under consultant care, but this consultant was so caring he aimed to be there for all staff.

I tried to be brave, but very soon the pain became unbearable. My midwife had been called away to assist with another delivery. The aim was for each labouring woman to have her own midwife throughout the whole labour, but this is not always possible.

I went to the desk to ask for help and there was another midwife sitting there who told me I was not in labour yet and I had a long way to go. This midwife was so dismissive and uncaring. Something else that stayed with me to take forward in my future practice. Listen to your birthing mother and always show compassion.

I went back to my room and was desperate for the pain to stop. Soon afterwards the night staff came on duty which I realised when there was a knock on the door and my next midwife introduced herself to say she was continuing my care.

On seeing my distress, she asked me to pop on the bed so she could examine me to see how I was progressing.

Her finding was that my baby was lying posteriorly, with the baby's back pressing against my spine causing the constant back pain. This midwife arranged effective pain relief and from then on, I had complete trust in her to take care of me and my unborn baby.

I felt safe in her hands simply because she had made me feel she cared. I will always remember that feeling and I still remember her to this day.

I went on to birth my baby with the help of forceps. I still needed to push while the doctor gently pulled and turned her round. Forceps are instruments that are applied to a baby's head to assist in delivering the baby.

My baby daughter, Emma, was put in my arms and my previous ordeal was forgotten. I felt completely overwhelmed with love for this beautiful little person and experienced the wonder of childbirth.

Emma now has her own family and has followed in my earlier footsteps as a nurse. She is a successful matron working at Harefield Hospital.

The birth of my second daughter Sally, was textbook, just as if I was in my antenatal class, doing my breathing exercises and in complete control.

I worried during this pregnancy that I might not feel as much love for my second baby. How wrong I was, I again felt as overwhelmed with love as I did with my first child. I went home on day two and introducing Sally to her older sister was just so exciting. There were so many special moments.

Sally had several health issues growing up and there were some challenging times. Sally spent time on various wards in several hospitals and my training came in handy when helping to care for her, especially when she was on the Orthopaedic ward.

As an adult, she still has some health issues, although this has not stopped her from fulfilling her dreams and she too has a family. She also followed in my footsteps joining the health care profession. Sally worked as a health care assistant on a children's ward for many years, using her own many experiences as a child in hospital, to support sick children and their families. At present she works in the preoperative screening and admission ward at Harefield Hospital.

Our third child, Lisa, joined us two years later, another girl to complete our happy family and again just as exciting. I experienced several hospital admissions for bleeding during this pregnancy and having two older children to consider meant there was some balancing of child-care. Thank goodness for family and friends.

On my last admission, I had been in for a few days when the consultant thought he should induce me and deliver me early, at thirty-six weeks. This happened very quickly in a side ward, not a birthing room with everything prepared. I felt I needed to go to the toilet to have my bowels opened and was told I had to use a bedpan. Like many other women I mistook this sensation, it was not like my first two deliveries. I would have thought by now I knew whether I was having a baby or a bowel movement, this time it was my baby's head presenting.

I rang the bell and a student midwife responded and just caught her as she arrived. The student midwife was lovely, and I was very impressed by her calmness and competence. I wrote a letter stating this to her tutor and she thanked me with a message of her own.

This experience showed that when nature takes over, there is very little you can do. When a baby wants to come, it just happens.

I was upset at the time, as because I was not in a proper birthing room Lisa was taken away to another room to keep her warm and I didn't hold her for about an hour.

Naturally I was stressed and worried that she was alright. Since then, although it is a priority to keep mother and baby together, I always made sure mothers who had just given birth were kept informed about their baby's whereabouts if they had to be separated.

A quick delivery is known as a 'precipitate labour', which is when a labour is very quick and short, and the baby is born less than three hours after the start of contractions.

Lisa had her two older siblings fussing and fighting over her and what she lacked in weight at just 2.2kgs, she made up for in spirit. Lisa was a healthy happy child who was very soon holding her own amongst her siblings. She also has her own family now.

Lisa did not follow in my footsteps in the medical profession, but like me has a love of horses and dogs. She has had a successful career caring for people in customer services for British Airways and currently works in Human Resources for a recruitment company.

I loved being pregnant and the whole experience of giving birth. My own births were all different and provided me with some valuable insight for my future practice, with an understanding that every experience is personal to each woman. With this, in mind I vowed always to keep an open mind and embrace any new birthing experiences as a learning opportunity.

I loved being a wife and mother and felt completely fulfilled. I felt there could be nothing better. I did not think then that I would find further fulfilment in my nursing career.   I initially returned to nursing to help the family finances.

THE NEXT STEPS

I returned to work part time, increasing my hours gradually. I was working as a State Enrolled Nurse in the same maternity unit at Northwick Park Hospital, where I had worked before having my children. I gained valuable experience while working amongst some brilliant midwives and observing their practice.

It was at Northwick Park Hospital, where I met Mary Kershaw, the ward Sister where I was working. Mary would become the driving force behind my decision to become a midwife. I remain to this day, eternally grateful to her for the faith she had in me and for the passion in midwifery she instilled in me. Mary understood the importance of my family life but helped me to see that with encouragement I could manage both.

In 1987, a conversion course was introduced to enable State Enrolled Nurses to upgrade and become State Registered Nurses.

I knew if I was able to enrol on this course and qualify, I might have a chance to go on and train as a midwife. I was very anxious and doubted my ability to be able to secure a place on the course. Mary literally took me by the hand one day and marched me to the office to apply.

It is her I have, to thank for achieving my dream of becoming a midwife and all the years that followed in a career I absolutely loved. Mary taught me so much and has remained a close friend to this day and I cannot thank her enough for what she did for me at that time.

Becoming a midwife was not going to be easy for me as I found out after a setback during the conversion course.

I will admit that studying and having a young family was a challenge. I had managed to get through the course until the final exams. However, I was never confident that I would pass despite everyone telling me they were sure I would pass and that I was worrying unnecessarily.

Imagine how disappointed I was when so close to success, I found out that I had been referred on one of my final papers. It was a day I will never forget. I knew it was going to be hard and passing was far from a formality for me and the result was devastating. I knew I could not give up, although it did cross my mind. I had to continue and retake with the next cohort six months later.

This I did and was successful on the second attempt becoming a State Registered Nurse (SRN) in 1988.

The experience of failing part of my final exam really knocked my confidence. I had taken a job at St Vincent's Orthopaedic Hospital as a State Enrolled Nurse while waiting to retake the final paper.

Once I had passed my paper and became qualified, I felt I needed to consolidate my practice as a State Registered Nurse, so I continued at St Vincent's, as a Staff Nurse, to gain experience and confidence.

After two years, I couldn't shake off the nagging voice that was calling me to become a midwife.

AT LAST

After gaining experience as a Registered Nurse, I applied for midwifery training at Northwick Park and to my delight I was accepted.

I was 40 at that time, my children were more independent, and I was not planning to have any more. I am sure these factors enabled the employers to see me positively as a person who could really commit to the training and the role of being a midwife.

During my training I was fortunate to gain valuable experience from several mature midwives whose instinctive practice and "hands on skills" were amazing. They trained during the days before scans and electronic monitoring, they rode bikes, provided continuity of care, and really knew their women and their families. Their hands were their most valuable tools.

The most useful piece of advice they gave me was that "childbirth is a normal process, treat everyone as normal, know the normal and any deviation from the normal will always stand out."

In my training, we each had to complete a case study, following one mother along her pregnancy journey, attending all her appointments, building a rapport and being on-call for her when she went into labour.

My case study was Angela, a first-time mother who was a little overweight but otherwise raised no clinical concerns.

Angela's pregnancy progressed well, and I was called one night to say she had been admitted into the labour ward. I attended immediately, supported by a midwife I had not met before, who encouraged me to manage the labour and birth under her supervision.

Angela was pleased to see a familiar face and I was introduced to her husband for the first time. Angela progressed well through all stages to a normal birth of a baby girl.

This was a positive experience for me which I could reflect on in my future career. I would soon find out that things did not always go so smoothly.

There was another birth during my training I will never forget, when I thought "that's it, I'll be struck off now and my dream is over!"

I had just delivered the baby with my mentor and needed to cut the umbilical cord which connects the baby to the placenta. All was going well until I cut the wrong side of the clamp next to the skin! My mentor grabbed the bleeding stump and asked me for another clamp, she was so calm and managed to re-clamp the small amount of stump remaining. The umbilical cord must be clamped in two places, it is then cut between the two clamps to prevent any blood loss. I had cut the cord before both clamps next to the baby which could have caused a sudden blood loss from the baby.

Once out of the room I shared my fears with my mentor, "had I ruined my potential career, and would I now not qualify?" She was so lovely and reassuring. She could see my obvious distress and offered the following words of support. "We can all make a mistake, and it was rectified immediately, with no adverse effect for the baby." She also said I would never do that again and how right she was. That lesson along with many others stayed with me throughout my career.

The mother was informed of the reason for such a short cord and the baby was observed closely for 48hours.

I knew the seriousness of my error. A baby can bleed out very quickly from cord trauma at delivery and despite my mentor assuring me the blood loss was minimal, I tormented myself throughout my two days off until I returned to work to find both the mother and baby were well and going home. I continued with her post-natal care until transferring her care to the health visitor.

As practising midwives, regardless of experience it is important to recognise the importance of always learning.

I am pleased to see that an open and honest culture exists in the National Health Service, which encourages growth and development from learning.

I often shared this experience when mentoring future student midwives.

Midwifery training provides the valuable groundwork, for a career in which your knowledge and experience is gained daily. Every woman and her birthing experience is individual to her.

You continually gain experience from mentors, role models, colleagues and most importantly from the women you care for. You must always listen to what women tell you and observe their varying behaviours. That is how your practice will develop.

QUALIFIED

When I finished my training and qualified as a midwife at Northwick Park Hospital, there were no posts available to apply for, so I applied and obtained a position as a midwife at Central Middlesex Hospital, which was one of the other training hospitals in the group. I needed to work to be able to practice and consolidate the valuable experience I had gained as a student.

Many of the labouring women in this unit did not have English as their first language and would often arrive in strong labour, acting instinctively as their bodies guided them. It was amazing and I learnt a lot from them.

I attended women who birthed on the floor, in toilets, often kneeling and adopting other positions they felt comfortable in. In the 1990's these alternative positions would have been considered quite unorthodox. I also learnt a lot about communication skills.

I have reflected on these experiences throughout my career and my aim was to always empower labouring women to be in control of their birth experience.

After just six months, I was looking to expand my practice and attended a water birth study day, at Hillingdon Maternity Unit where I was shown examples of birth in water and listened to the mother's and the midwives' perspectives. I really enjoyed the day and found the proposition of water birth fascinating.

The head of midwifery at Hillingdon encouraged me to attend for an informal visit and the next thing I knew I was applying for a position within her unit.

This was a big step for me, but I recognised that I could move on from the security of a maternity unit I felt comfortable in, to a unit offering some exciting concepts in midwifery care. I am pleased I took that leap of faith, and I remained at the Hillingdon Maternity Unit for twenty-one years until I retired in 2014.

MIDWIFERY TEAMS

A midwife can practice in a hospital or within the community setting which includes a woman's home. In hospital a midwife is part of a much larger team, where there is always support and guidance available.

When delivering at home, a midwife usually has a colleague with them or back up from the emergency services if required, which are all part of the community team.

During my years as a midwife, I gained vast experience. I spent most of my midwifery practice in the community setting with my base being at the hospital. I communicated closely with my colleagues in the unit and the community clinics or GP practices.

I started at Hillingdon Maternity Unit in a rotational post gaining experience in the antenatal, postnatal and delivery departments.

Hillingdon was piloting a concept of 'team midwifery' and after an unsuccessful first application to join the pilot team, my second application was successful, and I joined a team of six midwives.

The team cared for a caseload of women throughout the north of the Borough, before, during and after their births. They provided total care from confirmation of pregnancy to handing over to a health visitor when the baby was six weeks old.

Women usually had their first appointment with a midwife in their home, where the midwife would be able to establish a rapport, assess the home, meet other members of the woman's family, and identify any possible concerns. This resulted in really knowing your women well.

The women in the team could choose to birth either in the unit or in their own home. The team held coffee mornings for the women planning a homebirth, ensuring that all the midwives would be familiar to the woman, before birthing took place.

The aim of the team was that women would be attended by one of the team whom they had already met. The pilot was a great success, and more teams were then established covering larger areas of the Borough.

GAINING EXPERIENCE IN HOMEBIRTHS

Prior to joining the team of midwives, I made myself available to go on call with other midwives attending homebirths. This helped me to gain experience and see if I would be able to manage the challenging hours and give me an insight into birth at home.

I had never attended a homebirth before and wondered if the responsibility would prove too great. I attended two homebirths with two very experienced midwives, each with their own individual practice.

At the first homebirth, I arrived to be greeted by the midwife who welcomed me and explained the couple's wishes for their birth. They wanted everything kept quiet, with limited conversation and the woman's wish was to be completely naked.

They were happy for me to attend, and I knew I needed to be respectful of their wishes and observe quietly. The labouring woman and her partner were upstairs.

Home births generally tend to be more relaxed and natural, as the couple feel more comfortable in their own home.

It was a lovely experience and after the baby was born, both mother and partner were very animated and happy for conversation. It was their second baby and the same midwife had attended them previously. They obviously felt safe and comfortable with her resulting in the care they wanted.

This was my first involvement where the mother remained naked throughout. Later, I reflected on whether this was something the mother would have felt comfortable to do in a hospital setting. However, in the privacy of her own home it felt right for her.

Many women have a fear of being out of control and exposed when giving birth. They feel vulnerable and will often ask beforehand, "please make sure I keep my clothes on or keep me covered". I often discreetly reminded them of their request when they began removing their own clothing during their labour and birth.

Giving birth is an experience you cannot predict, if it is your first time you have no idea how it will be or indeed how you will feel at the time. This is when a midwife needs to be mindful, sensitive, and supportive of each woman's individual needs.

The second homebirth was very different with lots of chatting and a very bubbly midwife. Again, the midwife was known to the mother, having delivered her previous two babies at home and they had a great rapport. This was another positive example and as soon as the baby was born there was knocking on the bedroom door.

The midwife covered the woman appropriately and called, "come in". In burst the two older siblings onto the bed beside their mother, delighted with their new sister. A magical moment to observe, the joy and naturalness, of giving birth in familiar surroundings with those special people around them. It is so rewarding to be able to provide continuity of care and having an opportunity to really know the mother and their family.

Over the years I became more involved with homebirths, developing my skills and further enjoying my practice. I was able to commit to the on-calls and unsocial hours as my children had grown up and were leaving home.

I was also fortunate that my husband was supportive, although he did find warming up his own dinner a challenge to start with! Graham knew I loved my job, and he no longer had me complaining when he went off to play rugby every weekend.

When on call, I would always leave everything ready in case the phone rang. My clothes were laid out ready to pull on and the homebirth equipment was checked and packed. I loved being on call and enjoyed the feeling of the adrenaline rising, as I hurried to make sure I arrived promptly. Some babies were in a hurry, and I always wanted to get there in time to ensure the baby birthed safely and that it was a positive experience for everyone involved.

There was one occasion when I crept back to bed after being called out for only a few hours and my husband asked if the call had been a false alarm. I replied, "no, I only just arrived in time, the baby was born safely, and all went well." After the necessary checks I left the family happy and enjoying their new baby. It was such a positive and fulfilling experience all round and I got back to bed before daybreak, a rare experience on a night call.

Having worked in one of the first midwifery teams early on in my career, I gained increasing knowledge and skills within a supportive environment. My practice became more positive, I gained in confidence and really enjoyed being part of a team.

It was in the team that I met another wonderful midwife, Sally Dauncey, who became my main role-model. Sally is a special person whose practice was totally woman focused. I aimed to emulate her example in my own practice.

Sally was a team leader, who later progressed to being our Head of Midwifery. I learnt such valuable skills and knowledge from practicing alongside her. To observe her with women showed me that was how I wanted to practice. I have her to thank for the amazing experience I gained as a practicing midwife, her hands-on skills with women, their families, and colleagues alike, were and still are to this day, second to none. Although I am now retired, I am privileged to be able to call her a true friend.

The guidelines for homebirths in the community are that they are attended by two midwives and sometimes a student midwife.

There is always support for the midwife at a delivery, whether at home, from a colleague or the emergency services, or in the delivery suite where there are the labour ward staff on hand.

As the team pilot progressed and became more popular the number of teams grew, and our service became a little less personalised. There were occasions when I was on-call that I was covering the whole Borough for home births. This resulted in attending some women I might never have met before. My aim then was to always try and put the woman and her birthing partner at ease as quickly as possible, supporting them during the labour and birth enabling the whole experience to be a safe and positive one.

In the home environment I needed to be mindful and respectful when entering the woman's home. These homes varied from flats to mansions and sometimes in out of the way places. The women might be affluent or poor and disadvantaged, and there were many differing cultural influences to be aware of.

Sometimes women were in strong labour when I arrived, and events progressed quickly. The priority was always to reassure the woman and family, check the woman's history, observations and prepare for a safe birth. There is always a planned second midwife at homebirths but sometimes babies did not wait for their arrival, and I just had to do my best on my own.

Generally, if a baby is coming quickly, most of the time they will be born wherever they are, nature just gets on with it and birth happens. Every birth continued to be amazing.

PRIVILEGE

For me being a midwife was a huge privilege. To be involved in a family's most intimate and life changing experience and responsible for bringing new life safely into the world, is the most satisfying part of the role.

Each mother brings her own culture, concerns, and fears, entrusting herself and her unborn baby entirely to your capable hands.

Over the years, there are many births I will never forget, for many different reasons. I was fortunate to deliver some women on more than one occasion providing total care and continuity. On such occasions I was able to establish a good relationship with the women and their families and it has been a privilege to remain in touch with some of them to this day.

Over the years I have cared for many friends and colleagues during their pregnancies. It was especially rewarding to look after some of my daughter's friends, who I had known as young girls and then to be present as they became mothers.

To be involved with their care I was often required to be available in my own time. Fortunately, I was able to commit to this as I worked within a supportive team. We were all happy to provide cover for each other if required.

When I was on call, I loved it when my phone rang and was always full of enthusiasm and anxious to get to the woman quickly.

The following stories are just a snapshot of some of my many memories that I wish to share with you now.

The women in this book have been given fictional names.

PLANNED HOMEBIRTHS

My First Home Delivery

My first home delivery as the lead midwife was with my team leader, Sally, providing support as the second midwife. I wasn't due to start on the team until the following week but there were two homebirths happening at the same time and no one else available, so Sally asked me to attend one woman, Brenda, saying she would be there for the birth as well as supporting a student midwife with another woman who was in the early stages of labour with her first child.

Brenda was labouring with her second child and progressed quickly with my team leader managing to attend for the birth. Things got a little messy, as unfortunately Brenda experienced loose stools throughout her delivery (which can occasionally happen). This proved quite a challenge for me keeping the loose stools off the baby's face while assisting Brenda to birth in a kneeling position.

Ever the professional, I managed the situation as sensitively as possible reassuring her, that she was doing well.

I went on to birth Brenda's third baby at home. This time I had provided her total care throughout the pregnancy and had got to know her well.

Again, Brenda preferred to birth in a kneeling position which was her choice. She again experienced loose stools but at least this time I was prepared, and she wasn't concerned as I'd "seen it all before". Both her labours were well supported, and she birthed safely, building my confidence as a competent midwife.

I gained experience in home births and really enjoyed being an autonomous practitioner. Over the years I have attended many home births, meeting some amazing families who have played an important part in my working life and who I remember fondly.

My Next Door Neighbour

One of my early homebirths was my next-door neighbour Carol, who was expecting her second baby and under the care of the team I was working in. Carol really wanted to deliver at home and asked if I was around would I be able to look after her.

I was on a day off when she rang me to say she thought the baby was on the way. I was just doing my chores at home and happy to go round and assess her. She was only niggling and in the early stage, all checks were normal for both her and the baby and she was happy for me to leave her and pop back later.

I informed the labour ward that Carol planned to deliver at home and was in the latent stage of labour at present and would possibly birth later that day. I informed them I was happy to attend her and that I would ring for a second midwife and the equipment once her labour became active.

I checked Carol after a couple of hours and her labour was now progressing. I rang for my second midwife who arrived in good time with the equipment.

Carol progressed to a lovely calm birth of a second daughter weighing 4.2kgs, she was so happy to have given birth at home just as she had wanted, with her husband present and her mother downstairs with her older daughter, who was introduced to her baby sister immediately.

This was a lovely experience for me, as in the early stage I was able to continue my chores at home until the labour established and I even attended in my slippers.

I continued Carol's post birth care and as a bonus, I was able to watch the baby growing up. It was a very relaxing experience for us both and reinforced the normality of childbirth.

Being Available

Another time, I was called to provide support for a mother who was in labour with her fourth baby. This birth like her previous three, was planned to be at home. Donna was well known to me as I had been the second midwife and provided her post-birth care for her third child. I had got to know the family well and it was a happy reunion when she became pregnant with her fourth baby and was allocated to my caseload. Donna assured me this was her last pregnancy and we both laughed at this.

When Donna contacted the team to say she thought she was in labour, I was on a day off and providing emergency cover for homebirths only, as the team was short staffed. I visited Donna to assess her progress. On examining her I found she was not yet in active labour. Active labour is usually confirmed when the mother is contracting regularly, with contractions lasting 1-2 minutes, with dilatation of the cervix at more than 3 centimetres. The cervix is the neck of the womb and assessment is made by a digital internal examination.

All observations for her and the baby were normal, so I left Donna with my contact number, advising her to call again when her contractions became regular and lasting longer.

I decided to return to my original plans for my day off, which was to book a holiday. We had been searching for the right holiday for some time and having settled on the perfect place I returned to the travel agent to finalise the booking. I was just about to pay when my phone rang. Yes, it was Donna from earlier and she was now contracting regularly and strong.

This was her fourth birth, and I knew I needed to go immediately as she was likely to be quick. I arrived in time, and so did my second midwife. Donna progressed and birthed her baby safely within the hour.

The next day, I returned to the travel agents to complete my holiday payment. When they pulled up my details on the screen, it was documented that I had been called away to deliver a baby! They all wanted to know if it was a boy or a girl and had I made it in time? They were all delighted and agreed that I deserved a well-earned holiday.

A Night at the Opera

Whilst childbirth can be an intense experience, there can also be lighter moments. This was beautifully demonstrated when a colleague (she will know who she is) and I attended a first-time mother Emily, in labour planning to birth at home.
They were both musicians and we were treated to very enjoyable music throughout the labour.

My colleague and I both shared a love of the show, "Phantom of the Opera" and the relevance of this will become apparent shortly.

Emily progressed well until the second stage and then there was a delay. The second stage of labour is confirmed once the cervix is fully dilated to ten centimetres to allow the baby to birth through.

Following the guidelines there comes a point when a decision needs to be taken whether to transfer the woman into the unit to give birth. This is usually if there is a prolonged second stage or no progress.

We discussed this with the couple and agreed to give them another fifteen minutes before deciding. Ten minutes later, Emily began involuntarily pushing and we could see the baby's head was presenting and on its way.

My colleague and I looked at each other and sang, "Past the point of no return", from Phantom. Something we all laughed about later over a cup of tea once they were all comfortable and reflecting on their successful homebirth.

A Russian Mother

One winter afternoon, I was called to attend a
Russian woman, Fedora, at home. I had not met
Fedora previously and she appeared to speak very
little English. It was her first baby and I needed to
understand her wishes while providing safe care.
There was a companion with her who also spoke very
little English and remained very quiet throughout the
whole birth.

My colleague and I were offered a hot drink, which we
accepted to be polite, hoping this would encourage
communication and confidence between us.

Fedora did not want a lot of monitoring but agreed to
me listening to the baby's heart rate with a 'Pinard'
stethoscope (this looks like a trumpet and is a manual
instrument used for listening to the baby's heartbeat).
Fedora had no objection to me checking her blood
pressure and pulse regularly.

Occasionally Fedora did decline this monitoring, so
while I respected her wishes, I made sure I
documented everything. I then left her a short while,
before attempting to monitor her again.
Throughout the labour there was Russian pop music
playing loudly, the lights were dimmed, and there was
limited conversation. This was a very different

experience for us but obviously a familiar one for Fedora and a comfort to her.

It was not an easy labour for Fedora or myself due to the difficulties with communication and my concern over her lack of understanding.

My focus was on ensuring her labour progressed normally to a safe birth, whilst remaining mindful of respecting her wishes. The labour did progress normally to a safe and calm birth in her lounge.

As soon as the placenta was delivered, I checked both Fedora and her baby, congratulated her on her beautiful baby, then observed the baby having his first feed.

I began tidying up and getting ready to leave, when Fedora stood up with her baby, went to her bedroom, wrapped the baby snuggly, and put him in the crib, then settled herself in her bed shut her eyes and said, "sleep now". As far as she was concerned, we had been dismissed!

I left Fedora's paperwork with her companion, gave her my number and (with some gesticulating) advised her to ring if she had any problems. I would return to see them the next morning.

I made sure to inform the labour ward of the outcome and my concerns regarding language and understanding.

The next morning Fedora was up, dressed and much more receptive and communicative. In labour she had obviously retreated, choosing to focus inwardly as her way of coping.

Meeting the Criteria

It is a woman's right to choose where she has her baby. However, this choice should only be exercised following full and frank discussions about the risks and benefits of her choice. On occasions the wishes of the mother may not align with the medical professional's advice.

This was the case with a first-time mother Grace, who really wanted a homebirth but did not completely meet the criteria. Grace was under consultant care and had several appointments with the consultant where she was repeatedly advised to give birth in the hospital.

Eventually in the final trimester, (the last three months of pregnancy), a plan was made to commence labour at home and transfer into hospital if there was any delay or deviations from the normal with her or the baby's observations.

I was on-call when Grace's labour commenced, which was fortunate for both of us as I had been involved in a large proportion of her antenatal care and was fully aware of all the preceding discussions and plans for her delivery at home.
Her labour progressed normally, and she began involuntarily pushing. On assessing her I found that

her cervix was fully dilated, and the baby's head was presenting well. I reassured her she was ready to birth and to listen to her body when she felt the urge to push. This she was happy to do and soon started active pushing.

Grace was now in the second stage of labour. I began monitoring more closely, as instructed by the guidelines for observations in second stage. I soon recorded some shallow decelerations (this is when the baby's heart rate drops). These decelerations became more prolonged the more she pushed and indicated a possible concern.

The baby's head which was presenting, was only just visible. I informed her and her husband we would need to transfer to hospital and rang for an immediate blue light ambulance transfer.

I changed her position onto her left side to promote oxygen flow to the baby and provided her with continual reassurance.

Unfortunately, this did not improve the baby's heart rate and it became obvious the baby was in serious trouble. The head was advancing now but Grace was exhausted. I knew I could not simply sit and wait for the ambulance to arrive and the best way to help this baby was to get it birthed as quickly as possible.

I calmly and honestly informed her that her baby was in serious trouble, and that she needed to birth quickly so I could help her baby. She was amazing and we worked together enabling Grace to find the energy to birth her baby quickly.

For a moment there was relief as the baby was born, but this was quickly replaced with a surge of adrenaline as I was confronted with an unresponsive baby. My colleague and I began active resuscitation with vigorous massage, drying and stimulating the baby.

I commenced rescue breaths with the ambu-bag (medical equipment used at home for actively inflating the lungs). Three rescue breaths are given to initiate inflation of the baby's lungs. To my relief the baby responded and although obviously shocked, improved with facial oxygen support.

The reason for the baby's distress soon became apparent as there was a visible true knot in the cord, the cord was also short and had become tighter as the baby advanced. If Grace had not given birth as quickly as she did the outcome may have been different.
Knowing Grace and her partner, being honest and having her trust resulted positively on this occasion.

The ambulance arrived as the baby was delivering. I was grateful for their support, and we made the decision to transfer into the hospital so the baby could be checked and observed, as he had a low Apgar score at birth. The Apgar scoring system assesses the baby's colour, tone, heart rate, respiration, and irritability at 1, 5 and 10 minutes after birth. 10 is the top score.

Thankfully, both Grace and her baby recovered well and returned home after twelve hours.

I later debriefed Grace and her partner on their experience. They informed me, they were very grateful for all the care they received and expressed some guilt over their decision to persist with a home delivery.

I reassured them that a true knot in the cord is a rare occurrence and could not have been foreseen. I also reassured Grace that apart from the knot in the cord and the short length of the cord her labour had progressed normally at home. It was also her tremendous efforts to deliver her baby despite being exhausted which had resulted positively in my being able to give her baby the initial support he required.

A Challenging Homebirth

There was a particular home birth early in my career that provided a valuable positive learning experience, that stayed with me throughout my career.

I was coming to the end of my on-call with half an hour left and was preparing to hand over, to my team colleague when my mobile phone rang.

It was one of our homebirth mothers who was overdue and had rung in reporting that she felt strange! I said I would pop round to assess her and then report back to my colleague who was due to take over.

On arrival I found Holly, kneeling in a bath full of water, she said "I'm not sure if it's the baby starting but I feel strange". With that, she gave an expulsive push, and I could see that the head was advancing quickly.

I asked her husband to call my colleague to come now, I pulled the plug in the bath, opened the delivery pack, and put on my gloves. The face became visible with thick green meconium covering it (meconium is the baby's first bowel movement and if passed in the womb can indicate the baby is distressed). There was no evidence of any amniotic fluid (often referred to as waters). In this instance the thickness of the meconium indicated that the baby was in severe distress.

My heart was pounding with the realisation of this grave situation. I asked her husband to ring 999, for immediate blue light ambulance support. I grabbed the mouth suction kit from the delivery pack, and I attempted to clear the baby's mouth with suction, whilst just the face was visible.

However, this was to no avail and Holly had another convulsive contraction and the baby fell, lifeless into my hands in the empty bath, Holly remained kneeling in the bath.

The baby was pale and lifeless. I checked the cord and could not be sure, but thought I felt a faint pulse. I cut the cord and commenced active resuscitation of the baby on the bathroom floor with both parents quietly watching on.

I asked the father to make sure my colleague and the ambulance could get in when they arrived. The father said he had not called the ambulance (he was obviously in shock), so I calmly asked him to please do so and inform them that the baby is delivered and that I have commenced active resuscitation.

The mouth suction was not clearing the airway so I shook the baby upside down as vigorously and as safely as I could. I then attempted mouth to mouth breaths along with cardiac massage.

Very soon my colleague's feet appeared at the bathroom door, I could not look up but asked her to help with the resuscitation. Eventually the baby spluttered, and a plug of meconium came up. I was then able to see the chest rise when I blew into her mouth.

My colleague had brought the rest of the equipment and we used this to maintain oxygen input until the ambulance arrived. Once I was able, I informed the parents the baby had been born in very poor condition and would need to be transferred to hospital. They were very quiet and just let my colleague and I continue with resuscitating their baby.

The ambulance arrived, and I felt a huge wave of relief as I could hand over the oxygen support to them. Unfortunately, they informed me that they were not confident to administer to such a sick baby, so I continued. We left immediately in the first ambulance and informed the parents they were sending a second ambulance for them.

My colleague continued to care for Holly and her husband, she delivered the placenta which needed to be taken to be with the baby in the hospital, and then they waited for the second ambulance.

The baby was forty minutes old by the time we got to the maternity unit and her condition was assessed using the Apgar scoring system. She only scored five. When the paediatrician asked me the history, I could not speak, my mouth was so dry from the meconium I'd been in contact with while giving mouth to mouth support and the trauma of the whole experience.

The parents arrived shortly afterwards in the second ambulance. It then hit me that possibly I had resuscitated a baby who was so poorly she might have severe and life limiting disabilities. However, this would never be a decision for me to make and I would always do whatever I could to preserve a life.

The baby was so sick she required immediate transfer to another hospital for a process of cooling. This was a relatively new treatment which involved cooling a baby's core temperature, allowing the body to rest and hopefully recover. After the period of cooling, the baby is gradually returned to a normal temperature while the medical team could assess brain function and any possible damage.

I kept in close contact with the family anxious to hear how the baby was progressing. To everyone's amazement, the baby recovered well and progressed normally.

I am delighted to tell you that I hear from the family every Christmas, with a photograph and news of how their daughter is getting on. She is now at university and doing very well.

When I think back to that delivery, I think I was in the right place at the right time. I can still see that baby's face when I was giving mouth to mouth and praying for her to breath. From that day onwards, I always said a prayer on my way to a home birth, asking for guidance and support. My Christian faith has helped me through many difficult times, and I certainly believe divine intervention was present that day.

I believe this baby was meant to live and I feel privileged to have been a part of her successful outcome.

This event proved that all the training I had undergone to become a midwife had provided me with the necessary knowledge and skills needed in an emergency. Even without all the equipment, basic training can work.

This experience had a very positive effect on my future practice, providing me with increased confidence in my ability to practice safely.

A Moment of Fame

One of the mothers, Imogen, who was on our team's caseload was expecting her third baby and was planning a home birth. Imogen had birthed her second baby at home and was attended by a photographer who captured the event for a magazine article. This had proved a resounding success so once again Imogen decided to share her childbirth experience and organised to have her third birth filmed.

This birth was planned to be at home and when she rang to inform the team she was in labour, the on-call midwife was already with another woman in the labour ward. The midwife did not want to let Imogen down, so she rang me to see if I could attend. My team knew I was always happy to help if available and thankfully on this occasion I was.

I arrived within fifteen minutes as I knew Imogen usually birthed quickly. She appeared to be coping well and said she was just going to have a quick bath. I asked her if I could assess her first, which she agreed to. Imogen seemed calm and relaxed, and the photographer was also on her way. You can imagine the surprise when I examined her and found she was fully dilated and ready to birth.

There was no time to waste, I needed to prepare for the birth along with checking both Imogen's and the baby's observations. Imogen did her very best to hold on as she was anxious to wait for the photographer. To this day I don't know how she managed to wait.

The photographer arrived and Imogen advised her to get her camera out quickly. She then sat down on the floor against the couch and calmly birthed her baby. Imogen was soon surrounded by the other children and the whole experience was magical. The magazine article was published with a picture of the father cutting the cord surrounded by the older children.

Imogen later sent this photo to a magazine, which wanted photo examples of homebirths for the front cover of a new book on homebirth.

The photo was chosen and the first I knew about it was when a colleague brought a copy of the book after recognising me. The photo showed me supporting her husband to cut the cord, we were on the floor with the older siblings watching on.

A Sibling's Understanding

I have been at several homebirths when the older children have been present. This can be a magical family experience, providing everyone is comfortable and the circumstances are appropriate, the birth can usually be managed with sensitivity.

A good example of this was Julie, who was due to have a homebirth with her second child. I received the call and was asked to go and assess her. I needed to examine Julie vaginally to assess her progress and I asked her if she was happy for her older child to be in the room. Julie replied to go ahead as her older child would not even notice, she was too busy playing. I proceeded to put on my gloves, and using obstetric cream I examined Julie as discreetly as I could.

Julie was not in active labour, so I left her with my number and advised her to ring again when her labour established.

Julie rang after a few hours and her contractions were now regular and strong. I called a second midwife and returned immediately. Julie birthed very quickly and gave birth calmly to a second healthy baby.

Later when I had packed up the equipment and was preparing to leave, Julie told me what her daughter had done after I left earlier.

Apparently, the little girl went to the kitchen, fetched the fairy liquid and a rubber glove, and asked her mummy to lie down. This just shows that however young a child might be, how aware they can be of what is happening around them.

A Woman's Control

As human beings there are situations where we may unexpectedly feel we have control over our bodies and indeed sometimes we certainly seem to.

This was clearly demonstrated by Kate, one of the women on my caseload who had planned a home birth for her second child.

I had provided the majority, of her antenatal care and we had established a good rapport. Therefore, I was delighted to be available when she rang in reporting regular contractions, and I attended quickly.

On arrival I found Kate in the kitchen holding onto the worktop, obviously in what appeared to be strong labour. I said I had better assess her progress, to which Kate asked if I could just wait until her mother arrived to take her older child away, she would be there very soon.

I was happy to wait and meanwhile listened to the baby's heartbeat and checked Kate's pulse and blood pressure. I could see she was progressing and was reassured that all was well with her and the baby.

I prepared for delivery while waiting and shortly afterwards Granny arrived, and her older child left happily with Granny. I think Granny could sense the urgency and appeared reassured when I advised her it shouldn't be too long.

I returned to the kitchen having said goodbye to her mother and older child, ready to escort Kate to be examined. With a sigh of relief, she said "no time".

I quickly prepared the area, and she sat down giving birth naturally on the kitchen floor. It was a beautiful birth and big sister soon returned with Granny to meet her new sibling.

Mother nature is amazing, that baby was ready to be born but Kate was able to wait until she felt reassured that her older child was safely looked after, she was in complete control of her body.

What No Knickers?

A colleague reminded me of one of her deliveries when she called me as her second midwife and to come quickly. She thought this story should be in my book.

I made it just in time for Ann's birth. Ideally there are two midwives at all homebirths, but sometimes a baby will not wait.

On this occasion I just made it in time and afterwards when everything was complete and everyone settled, I shared with them the information that in my haste, I did not stop to put my knickers on! I just threw on a track suit.

I was the lead midwife at Ann's next homebirth and this time I called the same colleague to be my second midwife.

The first thing she asked when she arrived, was "did I have my knickers on this time?" I reassured her and Ann that I had, and we all laughed.

WATERBIRTHS

The Best Laid Plans

It became apparent to midwives, that women often progressed quickly when using their bath for pain relief in labour, resulting in many women birthing unplanned, in their baths.

This prompted a guideline and training for midwives to assist birthing in water at home as well as in hospital. The guideline recommended that a suitable birthing pool should be used or hired if planning a home waterbirth. As with all homebirths, checks are made to ensure the home is suitable and the parents or supporters are fully aware of the guidelines.

Midwives have regular training and updates on waterbirths. It was at one of these study days that I was first introduced to Hillingdon Maternity unit and its forward thinking towards women's choices in labour.

I was on call and called out for Lorna's second labour at home. Lorna did not plan to birth in water but was using her bath for pain relief. There was no heat in the home, it was winter the house was quite cold, but the bathroom was warm and there was plenty of hot water. Lorna was happy in her bath and as the bathroom was the only warm room it was planned to birth there either in the bath or on the bathroom floor.

My colleague and myself discussed fully with Lorna what to expect if she happened to be unable to get out of the bath, resulting in her delivering in water.

Despite expressing a prior desire to get out of the bath to deliver, many women either change their minds at the last minute or some are simply unable to get out when they planned to.

When this happens, the midwife needs to ensure the water level stays above the baby's head so the baby will not take a breath until completely delivered.

Humans are born with an innate reflex that prevents a baby from breathing until they enter the air. If born in water the same reflex applies, providing the baby is not showing any signs of distress.

I have delivered many babies at home in water. There should always be discussions beforehand, so that women are fully prepared.

Lorna did not have a partner or anyone else with her and wanted her older child to be present at the delivery. However, although Lorna got to second stage of labour the baby took a while to advance. All observations were normal, so we let nature take its time. The older child became bored and asked if he could go out to play with his friends, Lorna was happy and agreed to this.

We suggested Lorna had a sweet drink and a banana which can often stimulate birthing. Her labour then progressed, and Lorna did not feel able to get out of the bath, but with my reassurance and guidance she safely progressed to a normal birth in her bath. Lorna's son came straight in to meet his sister once she was born, and the family were left happy at home.

As there was no heating in the home, Lorna was advised how to keep the baby extra warm and to encourage a further feed. I called later that evening to check on them both and was delighted to find that they were both doing well.

Not everyone lives in ideal conditions for a home birth, but providing plans are made most situations can be managed safely.

First Time Mother

Mary was a first-time mother on my caseload who had planned a home waterbirth and had hired a pool in readiness. I had seen Mary regularly during her pregnancy and we had developed a good rapport. I was on duty when she went into labour, and I really looked forward to helping her safely birth her baby.

The couple were very excited and had everything prepared with the pool set up in the lounge.

The labour progressed well and during our chatting we discussed the baby's expected gender. They were informed at the scan that they were expecting a baby boy. I reminded them that they were also advised there was always a margin of error and a possibility the scan may have got it wrong.

Little did we know then, that as I helped guide their baby up out of the water, into their arms, it was to meet their baby girl!

It did not spoil the moment and we laughed about it afterwards. They were amazed by the whole experience of meeting their baby and were delighted regardless of the gender.

They had achieved the perfect, calm experience and birthed their baby the way they had planned, in a pool at home.

A Full Conservatory

When attending a homebirth, it is important to remember as a midwife, you are a guest in that home. You are there to support the woman's wishes as far as possible, while ensuring you use your expertise and experience to safely bring their baby into the world.

I attended another home water birth where the pool had been set up in the conservatory. The conservatory was fairly crowded as Nicola wanted her children, her mother, an aunt, and the family dog with her.

I set up my equipment and ensured I could always maintain access to Nicola. Everyone worked well together, and Nicola's labour progressed as she had wanted.

Nicola was a serving police officer who patrolled in the police helicopters. Apparently, she had forbidden her colleagues to fly overhead that night, due to her planning to birth in her glass conservatory.

It doesn't really matter who is present at a birth, providing the mother's wishes are respected safely. If having the family pet present promotes a positive experience for her, then that can be accommodated.

Of course, the attending midwife needs to be comfortable with a dog and whoever else is present along with being confident they are able to practice safely.

Nicola had the birth she had planned and was very happy. I could normally accommodate a woman's wishes and thus hopefully promote a relaxed, positive experience for all involved.

Big is not Always Best

On another occasion, I attended a homebirth where Olivia and her husband had decided on a waterbirth for their second birth. They had birthed in their bath last time and this time planned to be organised and hired a pool.

When I arrived, the pool was set up and ready. It was a super-duper, all singing and dancing pool, which incidentally was really, too big for the room and overly too big for giving birth in as it was hard to get close to her.

The room had soft lighting with Nicola's choice of relaxing music playing. The labour progressed normally, and everything went well until the baby birthed behind the mother who was kneeling in the pool.

When a baby births in water it is usually guided gently up between the mother's legs, and into her arms.

If the baby births behind the mother, bringing it to the surface can be a problem if the cord is not long enough.

Nicola was still kneeling, but too far away in this enormous pool for me to reach her to guide the baby up safely. I had to put one leg in the pool, to reach down and guide the baby back through her legs so she could pick her baby up.

The biggest most expensive pools are not always the best.

This highlighted the importance of checking in advance the preparations made for a planned birth at home in water.

BBA'S
Born Before The Arrival Of A Professional

These deliveries are often the result of what is known as a precipitate labour, when the mother progresses very quickly before she can get to hospital or be attended by a professional.

When a woman or supporter rings to say the baby is coming quickly, a midwife or professional will offer advice and stay on the phone, while another midwife and ambulance are despatched. The professional on the phone will provide advice and support until a professional arrives.

When a baby is in a hurry, a midwife truly needs to be "With Woman," (which is the definition of what midwife means) using her skills to gain their confidence very quickly.

Sometimes you just need to help the woman to focus, slow her breathing and allow her body to function naturally when she is birthing quickly. This usually results in a calm normal birth being achieved.

Blue Lights

In my usual rush to get to one BBA, I spotted an ambulance ahead with its lights on which seemed to be heading in the same direction. I followed the ambulance with blue lights flashing and was grateful when I realised, we were both heading for the same address.

I'm sure many midwives had often wished they had a blue light, when trying to arrive in time.

We arrived to find Paula, kneeling on her bed with her bottom in the air, as she had been advised over the phone, by a midwife on the labour ward.

The back of the baby's head was just visible, indicating the baby was presenting normally. Paula was shocked and not actively pushing, so all baseline checks were made on the mother and baby ensuring all observations were normal. This provided an opportunity to establish her history and build some sort of rapport with the couple.

Paula seemed to have shut down and the contractions had momentarily suspended. The ambulance crew were anxious seeing the visible presenting part and wanted to transfer her to hospital.

I reassured them that the baby's heart rate was good, the mother was now calm and that it might be safer to birth where she was.

I encouraged Paula to change position, and this had the desired effect.

Within minutes her contractions resumed, and she calmly gave birth to her baby in her own home.

I was able to check all was well with both the mother and baby, talk through her birth experience and leave the couple calm and content to remain at home.

Ambulance crews are amazing and sometimes the only professionals present at a BBA delivery. They also provide brilliant back up for homebirths if required.

There have been many occasions when I have been grateful for our ambulance service.

A Little Privacy Please

On another occasion I arrived at a large, gated property with two ambulances already in attendance. I was shown up to the bathroom where Rachel was lying on the floor looking shocked and lost having just birthed her baby. There were four paramedics standing over her waiting for the placenta to deliver.

I introduced myself to Rachel and her husband. I then briefly checked the baby who looked fine and was being kept warm by the father.

The bathroom was very crowded. I asked those in attendance if perhaps we could give Rachel some space so I could give her my full attention. The paramedics kindly left the room and a relative made tea for them all.

Rachel was overwhelmed by the whole experience. I reassured her she had done so well and that we just needed to deliver the placenta (afterbirth) and she could then be made comfortable and enjoy her baby. Rachel relaxed and the placenta delivered naturally, completing the third stage of her birth.

I informed the labour ward that the birth was complete and that they were happy to remain at home. The ambulances left thanking them for their tea, it had been a happy shout for them on this occasion.

All the post-birth checks for Rachel and her baby were completed and normal. I made sure feeding was established and gave the parents the contact numbers to get in touch with the midwifery team if they had any concerns. They would have a routine visit the following day.

I spent time talking through the whole experience with them both and once they were happy to be left, I took my leave of the family who were happy at home, recovering from the experience and enjoying their new baby.

Christmas Present

One Christmas Day, there was a call to the labour ward from a very anxious father who said he could see the baby's head.

The labour ward midwife stayed on the phone talking to the father, giving advice and reassurance, while another called me to attend the BBA.

The baby came so quickly taking them both by surprise. The father supported Susan and with the labour ward midwife's advice assisted with the birth of his baby. Meanwhile I made haste to get there.

All was well by the time I arrived, and I was greeted by the magical sight of them both, appearing a little shocked and sitting by the Christmas tree cuddling their new baby.

It was such a magical sight and with their consent I took a photo for them capturing the special moment.

Homebirths around Christmas time can provide a little extra magic. I have delivered several babies under or near the Christmas tree. A Christmas present they will never forget.

BBA's are an example of just how normal birth can be and how they can happen to anyone anywhere.

Ideally, we make plans and arrangements for the optimum outcome for our births, but we also need to be mindful that sometimes "mother nature" takes control.

HOMEBIRTH TRANSFERS

All midwives have guidelines to follow when delivering babies at home.

If there are any concerns or delay during a homebirth an ambulance is called to transfer the woman to hospital. The midwife always transfers with the woman and whenever possible the birthing partner goes too.

This is an unusual outcome as most homebirths are successfully completed at home.

Bus Stop Births

On two separate occasions I have delivered a baby in an ambulance, at the same bus stop. This bus stop was at the beginning of the road leading to the hospital.

The first occasion was a delivery where there was a delay in the second stage and following the guidelines to ensure an optimum outcome for both the mother and baby, I advised her to transfer so she could give birth in the hospital.

Typically, once on route to the hospital, nature took over and this baby decided to arrive after all. I informed the crew we may have to pull over, the response was "hang on we're nearly there".
My response was "pull over now" and I just caught the baby.

The baby delivered safely, and we continued onto the hospital. The crew were particularly happy as they could have an extended break, while they cleaned and re-sterilised the ambulance.

On the second occasion it was a similar situation, a different crew but the same discussion about pulling over immediately. This birth happened at the same bus stop and safely in the ambulance.

However, this couple took great pleasure in informing everyone they knew that they had delivered their baby at a bus stop.

I did advise them, to explain that although they had given birth at a bus stop, they were in the safety of an ambulance with their midwife!

HOSPITAL BIRTHS

Quick Is Not Always Best

I had just completed a twelve-hour shift on the labour ward and was saying goodnight to a colleague at the desk when the doors opened and a midwife from upstairs entered, pushing a woman in a wheelchair who was obviously in strong labour accompanied by her partner.

Davina was requesting a waterbirth. The response from my colleague at the desk was that this was not going to be possible tonight, as she had just received several calls from labouring women who were on their way in and would be arriving imminently. The labour ward was short staffed, as they had not managed to get agency cover and were one midwife down.

Davina was crestfallen, and I appealed to my colleague. Her response was, "if you would like to stay and look after her, she can have a waterbirth". My conscience got the better of me. Davina looked to be in strong labour and would probably deliver quickly so I would not be too late home.

Davina was delighted and progressed well, giving birth quickly in the pool as she had wanted.

They were a lovely couple, and I was so pleased to have been able to facilitate this special experience for them.

I had completed everything and checked they were both recovering well. I was then going to hand her care over to the labour ward staff who would continue her care and arrange her transfer to the ward.

However, on checking her blood pressure, I found it slightly elevated from her previous recordings. Davina also informed me she was feeling some discomfort down below in her perineal area. I rechecked her perineum which is the area between the vagina and anus where I found she now had a small haematoma, which is a collection of blood.

There were no signs of a tear or trauma to the perineum. I handed these observations to my colleague who reassured me she would continue to monitor her and advised me to go home.

The next morning, I went in to find that Davina had required surgery, to have the haematoma drained as it continued to increase in size. This was likely due to her high blood pressure which had continued to rise, resulting in eclampsia, a serious condition in pregnancy which can occur very quickly.

This was a probable explanation for her quick delivery, which can happen when the body tries to protect the unborn baby from the stresses of the impending eclampsia.

Obviously, the experience left the couple in shock, particularly when they were made aware of the eclampsia and the potential severity of the condition. Davina's pregnancy had been normal up to going into labour.

I stayed in touch with the couple, continuing their follow-up care once home. I often reflected on that experience, which made me aware that a quick birth is not always the best and could possibly be indicative of an underlying issue.

Adverse Effects of Analgesia

I have many experiences of labouring women, all of which are unique. There are always some women, I will always remember.

It was Eve's fifth birth. I had attended her twice previously and was familiar with her unusual reaction to Entonox analgesia, sometimes known as laughing gas.

In Eve's case she became a little bizarre acting totally out of character, she would suddenly glare at you angrily and stop communicating. I just managed her sensitively and helped her birth her baby. Once the Entonox was stopped, she soon returned back to her normal self.

Entonox is a self-administered, effective, and non-invasive method of pain relief which does not cross the placenta so does not affect the baby. Although it is only short lived, some women can have an adverse reaction which was the case with Eve's previous experience.

For this reason, she was not keen to use Entonox. However, she was progressing quickly and in strong labour needing some immediate support. We discussed using the Entonox again for immediate effect, as it did not look like she would be long before she birthed.

Eve agreed to try a little Entonox to help her progress. The Entonox was used, and she progressed quickly to another normal birth.

Once Eve stopped the Entonox it was immediately out of her system, and she was back to her normal self and able to enjoy her baby.

Keeping an Open Mind

All women are individual when giving birth, they cannot necessarily anticipate what their experience of childbirth will be. It is usually different for each woman and each birth. Women need encouragement and reassurance to have confidence in their body and its ability to birth their baby.

Even when supporting women in their choices for giving birth, not everyone is able to birth without some help from their midwife and sometimes further assistance is required from an obstetrician. They should be given as much information as possible and reassured that if there are any difficulties there will nearly always be help available.

Occasionally, I came across a pregnant woman totally focussed on doing everything naturally themselves and this was the case for Fiona, who was determined to stay home in the early stages of labour and have as little intervention as possible.

It was Fiona's first pregnancy and I attended her at home in labour. On examination her cervix (neck of the womb) was three centimetres dilated and she was contracting regularly.

Fiona met the criteria to remain at home, she appeared to be in active labour and was coping well. When I next assessed her progress there was no change internally and she remained in the latent stage of labour.

Latent labour is when the cervix becomes soft, thin and starts opening for the baby to be born. This can take hours or sometimes days. Fiona's internal assessment met the criteria for active labour, but she was not progressing.

Analgesia was offered but she was very focused on wanting to deliver normally without any pain relief. After several hours with no progress and still declining pain relief I advised Fiona, we should go into the unit.

Feeling disheartened and tired, she agreed, and we made our way to the maternity unit. Once there I again offered her analgesia and she tried some Entonox (gas and air), but she didn't get on with this as it made her feel sick.

Fiona agreed to try an injection which would not affect the baby, this was administered but there still was no progress. Fiona continued to contract regularly coping with the continual pain. An epidural was discussed, as by now Fiona was exhausted. This time she agreed to have the epidural and the anaesthetist was asked to attend.

An epidural is a procedure that injects a local anaesthetic into the space around the spinal nerves in the lower back. The anaesthetic usually blocks pain from the labour contractions during birth very effectively. With an epidural a mother can usually still push her baby out when she is ready to.

Within an hour the epidural had the desired effect resulting in Fiona getting to full dilation and progressing quickly to the normal birth she had always wanted.

This example shows us that sometimes we can become so focused on doing everything naturally, that we limit our body's ability to let go. In this example the effective analgesia had the desired effect, allowing Fiona's body to respond and progress.

I looked after Fiona in her second pregnancy and was again on-call to deliver her. This time Fiona came straight into the unit asking for the epidural.

I performed the physical examination to assess the progress of her labour, she was already 6cm dilated and obviously in active labour this time and should deliver very soon.

Fiona still wanted the epidural as she did not have confidence that she could deliver without it remembering her last birth. I did not want to deny her and inhibit her progress again, so I offered her an alternative method while waiting for the anaesthetist to arrive and site the epidural.

The injection was given with her consent allowing Fiona to relax and progress. Within minutes she began involuntary pushing and went on to birth normally without the epidural.

Both births were very different and provided valuable examples of the workings of childbirth, highlighting that each birth is individual, along with each mother's choices.

The workings of the human body always continued to amaze me.

Respect and Listen to Your Woman

I met a lovely Irish woman, Tania, during her first pregnancy. She was bubbly and enchanting in her manner and was also very clear what she did and did not want for her pregnancy and birth.

Tania advised me in a forthright manner that she intended to have every intervention possible and all available pain relief. She was also very clear that she would not be breast feeding, and requested politely but assertively for me, "not to discuss it further". I reassured her that her wishes were documented and that it was not a problem.

On the night she laboured I was due to relieve a colleague at midnight. My colleague rang me to say that she would like to stay with Tania until the baby was born as all was going so well and that Tania was in the pool!

At 0200 hours I had another call from my colleague to say things were not progressing so well now and could I please come in to continue Tania's care. I was happy to do so and duly arrived to take over from my colleague. Tania was now out of the pool due to the slow progress.

The labour eventually concluded in a traumatic forceps birth of a baby boy. The baby required support and was transferred to the neonatal unit. The parents were both in shock and very distressed.

I supported them throughout and was very concerned for them all. I went back first thing in the morning to check on them and see how they were.

I will never forget the sight that greeted me the next morning. I walked into their room to find Tania with her son, and she was breast feeding! It was a sight I will always remember, especially in view of her having been adamant that she was not going to breast feed.

I said I was so pleased they were both well and especially, to see her breast feeding. Her reply was "the poor wee thing, what he went through. When they brought him to me, I just took him in my arms and he turned towards me, so what else could I do?".

Tania had become a mother, which was another valuable learning experience for me. It is so important to actively listen to your woman, respect her choices, and remember that she like all of us, is entitled to change her mind. How does a woman know how she will feel when her baby is born?

I later cared for Tania in her second pregnancy, she was very anxious remembering her first experience. I offered to call round to her home and debrief her and her husband on their first birth.

During the discussion Tania informed me she had not felt listened to during her first birthing experience. She had been in the pool for pain relief but had not wanted to deliver in the water. Tania had felt her 'waters' pop while she was in the pool and wanted to get out, but the midwife had advised her that she was mistaken, and her waters had not ruptured. The midwife advised her that she was doing so well she would be advised to stay in the pool.

From then on, her first labour had not progressed, and Tania believed this was because she had been aware her delivery was imminent, and that she had not wanted to deliver in the water.

The midwife who attended Tania at the beginning of her first labour, later reflected and recognised that she should have listened to what Tania had been saying and what she had originally wanted. Listening to your woman is such a crucial part of being a good healthcare professional.

I agreed to provide all Tania's care during this second pregnancy and to hopefully be available, putting myself on-call for her, to ensure she would be listened to this time.

It was early on a Sunday morning, when I received the call to attend Tania at home to assess if she was in labour. The intention was to assess her and when suitable transfer in with her to the labour ward and support her through her birth.

On examination all was normal but she was already in advanced strong labour and dilated to six centimetres. It looked like Tania would give birth very soon, and I was not happy to transfer at this stage.

I explained the situation fully and reassured her that I felt it would be safer to stay put and give birth at home. With her agreement I promptly called for a second midwife and prepared to birth at home.

The whole birth progressed well, with the safe arrival of a baby girl, a sister for the older brother. It was a lovely calm delivery on the floor of their lounge next to the fireplace.

Both births were totally different which is often what happens when the first birth is difficult the next birth can be so different and sometimes much quicker.

When the couple reflected on their recent birth, they said they had found the whole experience a very positive one. Once all the post birth checks were complete and the baby had fed, I left the family safe and happy at home.

In the future when Tania looked at the fireplace, she told me that she would well up with emotion at remembering such a magical experience.

Building a rapport with Tania and her husband, listening to their fears and being there for them made such a difference. Another valuable experience for all involved.

Happy New Year

I had a photo taken of me, one New Year's Eve on the labour ward, having just delivered a baby with me wearing a sparkly top. An unusual birth photo for the family album, but hopefully a happy memory for that couple.

By way of explanation, I will explain. I should have been off duty and planned to celebrate the New Year with my family. Due to sickness, there was no cover for our team from midnight.

I was contacted and agreed to cover once I had seen the New Year in. The labour ward said they would cover for the team if one of our mothers came in until I could get there after midnight. Obviously, there was no champagne toast for me that New Year.

I received a call to inform me that one of the women under our team's care had called and was on her way into the labour ward. I arrived by half past midnight and relieved the labour ward midwife who had been overseeing Una until I arrived, while caring for another woman.

I was delighted to see Una, who was on my caseload, and I knew her well. Una was progressing and looked like she would deliver soon so I grabbed some scrubs to change into.

However, before I could leave the room she started pushing, and everything happened so quickly I just could not leave her to change. Hence, they have a photo of me lifting their daughter into their arms in my sparkly top.

Premature Twins

I cared for one of my daughter's friends, Vera, in her first pregnancy. I provided total care for her which resulted in a lovely waterbirth with her first baby.

In her second pregnancy, Vera was expecting twins which meant she required consultant care. Despite this I kept in touch throughout her pregnancy, offering support and reassurance.

All was going well until one evening, when I received a call from a colleague advising me that Vera had been admitted at 28 weeks, unwell with what looked like pre-eclampsia.

If untreated it can become very serious resulting in eclampsia which is very dangerous when the mother can develop seizures or a coma.

Pre-eclampsia is a condition that causes high blood pressure in pregnancy with protein in the urine.

I went to the hospital immediately and by the time I arrived Vera had been taken in for an emergency caesarean section.

This is when babies are delivered surgically by an operation in the lower part of a woman's abdomen.

Due to their prematurity, both babies were transferred to the neonatal unit. The parents were both very shocked and scared as everything was so different from their first birth.

Vera was very unwell with the eclampsia. I stayed with her offering what support I could while her husband, went to see the babies once they had been stabilised on the neonatal unit.

Vera shared her fears with me, not only for her babies but for her own mortality, she reflected on how ill she felt and her concerns that she might die, she was very scared.

I felt humbled and was reminded of the impact that such events have on a family, from something that can be part of a midwife's day to day work.

The babies remained in the neonatal unit until they were fit and old enough to go home. Vera went home once she had recovered enough, visiting her babies during the day then going home at night to her older child.

There was a lot of organising to do but luckily, they had good family support, and everyone pulled together.

It's at times like this when family and friends are so important.

An Experienced Mother

Each birth is individual and special to that family. This was beautifully demonstrated by a mother on my caseload who was expecting her sixth baby. Wendy was a nurse herself and I had seen her in my clinic earlier that day. She was full term (40 weeks), and all her checks were normal.

Later that night I was called in to the unit as she was in labour. I was pleased to look after her and all was progressing well.

Wendy was kneeling on the bed as the baby began to birth, she put her hands down and lifted the baby into her arms herself, saying "my baby, my baby".

I moved aside allowing her to do this and it was the most moving sight and one that has always stayed with me. If not only to see Wendy help her own baby into the world, but it was her sixth birth, and she was as excited as if it were her first.

I continued her care at home meeting the whole family. They lived in a small, terraced house, which was homely, full of love and very organised. The children were very excited and so happy to meet their new sibling.

I met Wendy some years later, when she told me her eldest daughter was training as a midwife. I am sure she shared her mother's love of childbirth and was inspired by experiencing the joy of her mother giving birth six times.

A Woman's Wish

One of my roles, was to be involved in helping women to make plans for their births or debriefing them following a difficult experience.

On one occasion a colleague asked me to visit a woman she was discharging from the labour ward after a false alarm of being in labour. Yolanda had informed my colleague that she had really wanted a homebirth, but her GP had refused her request.

My colleague asked me if I could visit Yolanda with a view to assessing if it would be possible for her to have a homebirth at this late stage.

I visited Yolanda and her husband that afternoon and was greeted by a lovely couple. I explained that it was very late in the day to arrange a planned homebirth, but not impossible.

There was a homebirth list for all midwives on-call, informing them which births were due and where they were so the midwives could familiarise themselves with the location and any possible issues on access or parking, they might encounter.

Yolanda was anxious about going against her GP. I reassured her that her GP was not required to attend or be involved in their homebirth as the hospital would take responsibility.

They really wanted to go ahead so I went through the paperwork, and necessary preparations, then we made their plan for when she was in active labour. The plan was to deliver in the bedroom, their only concern was if she soiled the new white carpet which they had only just had fitted.

I then returned to the unit and added Yolanda to the homebirth list, informing each team of the late addition and where she lived.

Later that evening Yolanda called in to the labour ward to say she was sure she was now in active labour. Lucky for me I was on-call and really pleased to attend. They were obviously reassured to see a familiar face and this time she was in active labour. Preparations were made to protect the white carpet.

Yolanda progressed well at home and when she wanted to go to the toilet, I laid a trail of towels across the carpet just in case her waters broke. When she got to the toilet, her waters did break, and she wanted to push which was so normal and re-assuring.

We managed to get back to her prepared area by the bed without any leakage on the white carpet (something we laughed about afterwards) and Yolanda had the lovely home birth she had always wanted, just her and her husband, with myself and a colleague.

I continued all her post-birth care and was delighted to have been able to support them in their birth choice. Yolanda's GP was not happy and made her feel irresponsible, telling her that it could have gone so wrong.

Needless, to say they changed to another GP. Unfortunately, in the early days of my midwifery practice many GP's, did not have experience or confidence in homebirths. Once the hospital teams took responsibility, they were happy to be more supportive.

PREGNANCY LOSS

Sadly, not all pregnancies result in a live baby and a happy ever after. Families experiencing pregnancy loss, require the same care and support, with the added awareness and understanding of shattered dreams and expectations.

A baby's death does not only affect the parents, but the siblings, immediate family, and all those in their circle of friends.

There is no easy way to deal with the death of a baby and it relies on sensitivity and taking the lead from each parent's individual needs. This can be difficult as initially they may not know themselves what their needs are.

When I was working there was always a link midwife who specialised in pregnancy loss and to whom we could refer mothers whose babies had died.

A Devastating Outcome

I remember in my early years on the team, when one woman on my caseload, Bella, had come to the hospital with her partner. She had been admitted and they had been informed that their baby didn't have a heartbeat.

I went down to the labour ward to see them but felt I could not go in, as I was so devastated for them. A colleague found me and gave me some valuable advice. It is very upsetting for everyone, but it wasn't about me. I then went in, hugged them both and cried with them.

I listened to what they had been advised which was for Bella to birth normally through the vagina. Although awful to go through labour knowing the outcome, it would be better for her and her baby. Bella was reassured that she would have strong analgesia (pain-relief), to make sure she was pain free and as comfortable as possible.

They were both very scared but agreed to the advice. I asked if they would like me to be there for the delivery and they replied, "if I could it might help". It was arranged for me to be available, and I had good support from the labour ward staff.

During Bella's labour I sensitively discussed what to expect and what they thought they might wish to happen when their baby was born. Whether they might like to see or hold their baby?

Obviously, they were unsure as they did not know what to expect, they had never seen a dead baby before.

It was difficult to discuss in advance what the baby's condition might be at birth. It was not clear when the baby had died, so it was important to be honest and ensure they were adequately prepared.

In case the parents were not ready to see their baby immediately after it was born, I had a crib prepared where their baby would be laid.

A plan was made to have a sheet over Bella's legs during the birth. Once birthed I would cut the cord, wrap the baby, and assess the condition to better prepare the parents before asking them if they wanted to see their baby.

Bella was kept pain free, and the baby birthed normally. Thankfully I was able to reassure the parents their little girl was beautiful and just appeared to be asleep. They tentatively asked to see her, and Bella took her baby straight into her arms. I completed the delivery and made Bella comfortable. I then sat quietly in the corner completing the notes, while Bella and her husband spent time with their daughter.

After a while they asked if their parents could visit, and I made the necessary arrangements. I asked the couple if they wanted anything brought in for their little girl to be dressed in and perhaps her own blanket to wrap her in.

They agreed and I asked the grandparents for the requested items. I advised them to come in through the side entrance. I was mindful of their distress and the side entrance would be more discrete.

The grandparents arrived, were given tea, and allowed time alone with Bella, her husband, and their granddaughter. I left the call bell should they need me.

I later dressed their baby on Bella's lap, talking gently to the baby throughout. They later told me, it was such a comfort with me talking to their baby, it felt like she was a real baby! Which of course she was.

I continued their postnatal care which was extended beyond the standard ten days. Sadly, the postmortem found no cause for this baby to die in the womb, as is often the case and even more distressing. This can be particularly difficult to comprehend or come to terms with and this couple did not go on to have a further pregnancy.

Choices and Decisions

With another mother, I was reminded how each experience is so different and that as individuals everyone responds differently.

Carolyn's baby had also sadly died, near the end of her pregnancy. I provided her care in labour, and she progressed well to a normal birth. It was Carolyn's expressed wish that she did not want to see her baby.

I prepared a crib in the next room and carried the baby through there once birthed. I completed the delivery and made Carolyn as comfortable as possible. She was again offered the opportunity to see her baby, but she was adamant she did not want to, and her wishes were respected without judgement.

The father however, said he would like to see his son and Carolyn accepted his decision. I took him through to the other room and although he was obviously distraught, he spent some time with his son.

I could see how difficult it was for each of them, especially as they each handled it differently. Nevertheless, it is the role of the midwife to respect and support both parents.

It was apparent at delivery that the baby had a true knot in the cord. This is a rare occurrence and hopefully this knowledge provided an explanation and some comfort.

Carolyn was asked once more before her discharge, if she would like to see her son, but her decision remained unchanged, and this was respected.

I continued her postnatal care at home and accompanied the father to the baby's cremation, where there were just the three of us including the minister.

The couple went on to have two further babies. It was following the birth of their second child that Carolyn asked to see a photo of her first child. This was clearly the right time for her to address her feelings toward her first birth and hopefully this provided some comfort or closure for this mother.

Photos, foot, and handprints are always taken when a baby dies and if not requested by the parents, kept in the notes, should the parents change their mind in the future.

To lose a child is devastating and each family has their own way of dealing with it. Whether they do or do not want to see or hold their baby, it can also be very hard to leave their baby and go home without them. They may wish to have visitors and photos or just be on their own.

Over the years when visiting homes, I have seen some lovely photos on display of previous lost babies. A lost baby is never forgotten and can always have a place in the ongoing life of that family.

Some people might feel this is morbid, but at the end of the day, what is right for that family is what is important. Everyone has their own ideas on how loss should be dealt with, and it is a very individual decision for each family. Hopefully parents can be supported in a way that feels right for them.

When caring for women who have experienced previous loss, you need to be extra sensitive towards their possible fears of meeting this new baby. Although the birth of a healthy baby can be a comfort it can also bring mixed feelings, reminding them of what might have been and what they had lost.

Different Times

In the fifties, my mother lost her third child, my brother. In those days babies were kept in a nursery and only brought to the mother to feed. On the third day my mother felt there was something not quite right with her baby and that he was not feeding properly. My mother was not listened to, and no one checked her son.

When my father visited and raised her concerns with staff again, the baby was checked and found to be very poorly with rhesus incompatibility. This is a condition where antibodies in a pregnant woman's blood destroy her baby's blood cells. My father was told he might not survive and was asked if he wanted to have him baptised.

Only my father was present when my brother was baptised, as it was considered too distressing to even inform my mother, a decision made for her not with her and shortly afterwards he died. My mother never saw him again, not even to say goodbye. This was particularly difficult for my mother as she had not been listened to when she raised concerns about her baby.

It must have been very hard for my father, such a difficult experience for him, while supporting my mother and going home to two older children. As for my mother, not being able to see her baby again or say goodbye, it must have been devastating.

Following his death my mother went away to a nursing home to recover. It was only towards the end of her life and once I became a midwife that she felt she could share this experience with me.

Although the outcome may well have been the same for a sick baby in 1956, the circumstances surrounding his death could have been handled differently.

Thankfully progressive teaching has now resulted in there being sensitivity and compassion when dealing with a loss, accommodating the mother and the family's needs, and involving them all in decision making.

If a mother is Rhesus negative now, she'll be offered an anti-D injection to prevent her from making antibodies against her own baby due to the rhesus incompatibility.

THE MIDWIFE GRANNY

When my grandchildren heard I was writing this book they were fascinated to hear some of the stories and one of them asked if their births were featured.

I explained that the book was about babies I had delivered and my life as a midwife. I had been present at some of their births, but not as a midwife.

I thought about this afterwards and decided I could include my experience of their births as a mother, grandmother, supporter, and midwife. The latter a role I could never switch off from until I knew they had birthed safely.

I really wanted to be there for my girls, as my mother was for me, doing whatever I could to help. I was also mindful that they had partners, and I was their 'mother-in-law'! I always wanted to be there when needed but never to get in the way.

Over the years our family has grown, and no doubt will continue to grow further. After having three girls it was a joy and quite refreshing to experience 'son in laws', although catering for their bigger appetites at the Sunday roast, took a bit of getting used to.

During my training as a midwife, one son in law was particularly helpful with my academic writing. Another provided ongoing advice on everything IT. They all get along so well, and my husband is eternally grateful for some male company after a home full of females.

Working in the unit I was lucky that I was able to ensure my daughters received total midwifery care. Something I was able to provide for many of my women over the years and which gave me a great deal of job satisfaction.

My daughters were very fortunate that my role model and friend Sally, cared for them throughout six of their births and when she was not available for the last one, another wonderful midwife Laura, was able to attend.

On each occasion I trusted my colleagues would do their very best and felt happy to take a step back. This was a huge commitment on their part and greatly appreciated as it is not advised that you care for your own family.

My daughters were keen that I enjoyed a different role as a Grandmother. They also responded better to my colleague than they would have done for me!

I have seven grandchildren and each birth was memorable and special in its own way.

Oliver

My eldest daughter Emma wanted a home birth, something she had decided on long before she found herself pregnant. She based this on a traumatic experience during her labour ward allocation as a student nurse.

Emma spent most of her labour in her bath finding it helped with pain relief. I was kept occupied keeping a supply of hot water and feeding everyone.

After a while it became apparent that there was an issue with the hot water, so I resorted to carefully carrying up pans full of hot water. Health and safety would not permit a midwife doing this, so it was lucky I was there as a mother, and able to support my daughter's wish to remain comfortable in her bath.

I found this new role quite a challenge and as her labour was long, I decided to cook a roast dinner to keep myself occupied and make sure my friend and her student were well fed. They each came down one at a time to eat and afterwards my daughter said she had wondered where everyone was disappearing to. The second stage was taking a while and I knew they would be having conversations about transferring to hospital, when suddenly I heard my daughter come running down the stairs.

I thought she was going to run out of the front door, but she immediately ran back up the stairs saying, "I want to push". My colleague's expertise had the desired effect and within minutes I could hear her say "Oh my God!" as her son Oliver, was lifted into her arms.

It was such a relief and now I had to get used to my new role as a Grandma. It was the best feeling next to my own births.

Sophie

My next grandchild was a high risk, pregnancy under consultant care and again was managed by the same colleague, Sally. The labour was difficult and eventually resulted in an emergency caesarean.

I was with my second daughter Sally and her husband, supporting them in the anaesthetic room when suddenly her husband walked out. I was concerned that he was feeling squeamish or felt it was all too much for him but then after a short while he returned looking fine. On asking if he was OK, he replied that he was hungry and went to have a sandwich!

That is so typical of him, to this day he still needs feeding regularly. Our first granddaughter Sophie was gorgeous with a mop of auburn hair, and I was glad to be able to take precious photos for them of those special first moments.

Naomi

Our third grandchild was born again to our eldest daughter Emma who again had planned a homebirth. This time a pool had been hired and was set up in the lounge.

All was in place and ready with a plan that when she birthed, I would take the older sibling Oliver, to my other daughter's home nearby.

Emma rang to say that her waters had broken and Sally her midwife was on the way. I hurried over and when I arrived, I could see her labour was progressing quickly.

I suggested that her husband stay with Emma as it looked like her labour would be quicker this time and I would keep Oliver out of the way. Sally was on her way but had not yet arrived and my daughter asked me to wait until she was there because she felt things were very different this time.

Soon afterwards Sally arrived and asked Emma if she would like to pop upstairs to be examined. Emma sat down on the living room floor and said "no, here is fine". She was nearly fully dilated and on hearing this she almost dived into the birthing pool. Emma very soon delivered her daughter Naomi in the pool in their lounge. Naomi was a big baby and was a little shocked after the quick birth, she required active stimulation to take her first breath. It was a tense few minutes and I was glad not to have left with my grandson as the second midwife only just made it in time.

Naomi soon pinked up and then met her big brother Oliver. It was such a joy to see big brother welcome his new sister.

Grace
Then came grandchild number four. A first delivery for my youngest daughter Lisa, who also planned to birth at home. This grandchild was not in a hurry and went past her due date.

It was a beautiful sunny day when Lisa's labour began, and she coped well. The baby was estimated to be a good size and it took a lot of effort to birth her. I remember my colleague looking at me as she was birthing saying, "I think we might have underestimated her size", she just kept on coming. Grace weighed five kilograms, which was a good size for a first baby.

The birth went very well until the placenta would not deliver despite all efforts. Following the guidelines, an ambulance was called, and my daughter and her new baby were transferred to hospital.

Lisa lost a lot of blood, which is the risk when there is a delay in delivering the placenta to complete the birth. She had to go to the operating theatre to have the placenta removed manually. She was then reunited with her baby.

Following the lovely homebirth, unfortunately things changed, and the experience became quite traumatic. Fortunately, they were both home on day two when I was able to offer my support to help her recover. This I enjoyed as I did for all my girls.

Madeliene

Grandchild number five was my eldest daughter Emma's, third birth after two successful home deliveries.

This time she went past her due date and the baby was again estimated on the large size. This baby was not making an appearance anytime soon and at forty-two weeks my daughter was advised to go into the maternity unit to have her labour induced.

I remember how distraught she and her husband were, following two lovely home births and they had hoped for the same this time. I remained at home with their two other children Oliver and Naomi.

I was anxious for them both but was reassured by the fact that my friend Sally would be continuing her care in the hospital. I took the children out and brought two bunches of flowers, one pink and one blue to give to their mummy depending on what sex the baby was.

Sally admitted Emma to the water pool room, artificially broke her waters and, Emma got into the birthing pool. Everything was progressing well, and I received a call from my son in law to inform me that she was six centimetres dilated.

Remembering how quickly her last baby delivered, I told him he'd better go back into the room as the baby could deliver soon, and I would bring their older children to the hospital as they had planned.
I'm not sure why but I was crying on the way to the hospital and the grandchildren asked if I was alright? I reassured them I was fine and just very happy.

Years later they told me that in my haste to get to the hospital, I forgot to strap them into their car seats, something they had always remembered and luckily not told their parents. What a bad Grandma!

When we arrived, I gave them each a bunch of flowers and said if they had a brother give the blue bunch to mummy and the other to the midwife and if a girl the other way around. I sent them in and waited outside.

Emma was still in the pool and apparently in their excitement, they threw both bunches in the water. The baby, Madeliene weighed five kilograms and my daughter gave birth in the pool with no complications. Another successful birth and they were all back home after two hours.

Joshua

My second daughter Sally delivered her second child after eight years, she again had gestational diabetes which is a condition of pregnancy which required her to be managed with insulin injections and be under consultant care. Sally her midwife again provided her pregnancy care alongside the consultant.

The baby was estimated to be on the large size and in view of the previous emergency caesarean, an elective caesarean was planned. I did not go into the theatre with them this time as it was not an emergency as before, so I said I would wait in the recovery room.
Waiting to hear the first cry seemed like an eternity, which was a very different experience for me. I heard the cry then Sally came out and asked me to

put scrubs on and come into the theatre. There was no problem it was what they wanted.

I went in and they held up the baby for me to see, it looked the image of their first daughter, then they exposed his bits with such joy, they had a son.

Their daughter was brought up by her other Granny and I was able to take her in to meet her baby brother Joshua. Once again, a happy family photo.

Beatrice

My youngest daughter Lisa delivered her second baby six months later.

Following her previous home birth and admission for a retained placenta, she was advised to deliver in hospital. Although under consultant care she also had her own midwife providing full midwifery care.

Lisa was admitted two weeks past her dates for induction, which is when labour is augmented and started artificially.

I was in the room when her waters were broken, and her midwife asked me to get the registrar.

From that moment onwards everything happened very quickly. The baby's arm was presenting, and we were then rushing down the corridor to theatre for an emergency caesarean section.

My daughter was distraught after her previous home delivery and kept saying "I don't want a caesarean I don't want an epidural". We were trying to reassure her, but I think she was unaware of the seriousness of this situation and the presenting emergency.

Having managed to get the arm back inside the womb and the baby repositioned, the consultant was very understanding and as the baby's heart rate had settled, he agreed to a trial of vaginal delivery in the theatre.

An epidural was sited in preparation. However, then the baby's heart rate started dropping again so they proceeded with the caesarean section immediately to get the baby delivered safely.

I remained out of the way in the theatre and remember when they opened her womb, seeing this mop of dark hair in the distance and then there were arms everywhere. It was a difficult extraction as they had difficulty locating a presenting part.

It was a traumatic experience all round but luckily resulting in the safe birth of her second daughter Beatrice. I was very proud of my daughter, who after going through all that, as soon as she was in recovery, she asked for her baby and put her straight to her breast.

RETIREMENT

Throughout my career I have worked with some amazing colleagues, and clients alike. I loved being part of the team and I thank all my colleagues for their support and the amazing experiences we shared together over the years.

Every midwife brings her own approach and people skills to the profession. The same as each mother brings a different birth experience which is unique and special to her.

This is only a snapshot of my career. Please know that every woman I cared for was responsible for providing me with the excitement of what each day might bring.

I really loved my job. How many people can say they enjoyed going to work and sometimes being called out in the middle of the night? I always hoped that my women felt cared for and supported with their choices and birth experience.

I've had an amazing career, sharing my life and best accomplishments with Graham my husband, my three wonderful daughters, their partners, and our seven

grandchildren, who always have and continue to bring me endless happiness and pride.
Having been part of their lives from the beginning and now seeing them grow and finding their own way in life brings endless joy, I feel very blessed.

When I retired, things were changing greatly in the maternity services. Like nursing there is a shortage of midwives and less attractive training opportunities. This is a real concern, as every baby deserves the optimum start in life. Ideally with one to one, care in labour.

I recently met a student midwife at my granddaughters 21st birthday party. It was such a pleasure talking to her friend and hearing her passion and enthusiasm for midwifery, which reminded me of how I always felt. This was so encouraging and reassuring. I wish her and all midwives a happy and fulfilling career.

I was fortunate to have had the experience I did and on reflection, my fulfilment has enabled me to now, fully enjoy my retirement.

This is now my time with Graham, to continue enjoying our family, our dog, our friends, and our garden. We brought Poppy, an apricot Schnoodle puppy when I retired, a new baby to give me someone to love and ensure I kept fit and healthy.

ACKNOWLEDGMENTS

I want to express my gratitude to all the people who have made this book a reality.

My late parents whose example and support of family life, set me on my pathway in life and my chosen career.

Mary Kershaw, the ward sister I worked for as a State Enrolled Nurse. Observing her with expectant mothers, her hands on skills and experience were a lifelong example for me. She showed me the magic of childbirth. I am eternally grateful to Mary who set me on the pathway towards an amazing career.

Sally Dauncey, an amazing midwife, colleague, manager, and now life-long friend. Observing how she was with women, I knew if I could aim to be a fraction as good as her, I would find fulfilment in my career. I have had amazing experience and support from Sally, and she has been my main role model.

All the wonderful midwives I have worked alongside and learnt from. Every mother I have cared for, who has played a part in my being the "Midwife in Me" and the fulfilment my career has given to me.

I had once mentioned to a neighbour, Moira Smith, that I wanted to write a book about my life as a midwife. I made a start but did not get very far. It was six years later when Moira asked me about my book, that I told her I had not continued with it. She asked me why not as she would have loved to read it. I replied that I did not know if I could remember enough now. Moira said that was a shame and suggested it might give me something to do during the Covid lockdown?

I thought about it, and I certainly needed a project to keep me occupied when the weather was too bad to get in the garden, so I made a start. I thought I could not remember much but once I started the stories came flooding back and I really enjoyed writing this book.

Then of course to my husband and family, who have always been there, supporting me and putting up with the training, the unsocial hours and for me disappearing when the phone rang.

A special thank you to another dear friend Catherine Fahy, for proof reading, editorial assistance in publishing this book and the many hours spent supporting me throughout this venture.

I have enjoyed writing this book and now this is completed, I can start a new project.

Keep a look out for my next publication which could be a children's book.

Have You Seen Poppy Doodles?

Printed in Great Britain
by Amazon